This Journal Belongs to:

_____

This Journal is From:

_____

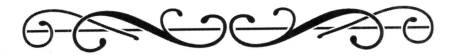

How to Use This Journal:

- Use it in your practice to write down reminders of things you need to do.
- Use it to journal your thoughts, and let your mind unwind at the end of a busy workday.
- Take it on a trip or vacation, and record your excursions.
- Record things your children or other family members are up to, so that you can reflect on everything, in years to come.
- Use your imagination!

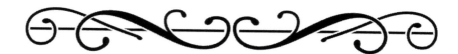

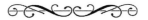

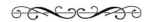

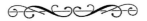

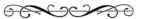

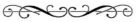

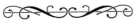

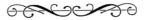

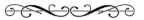

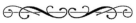

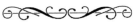

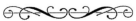

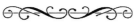

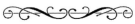

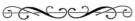

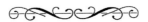

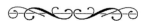

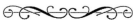

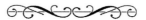

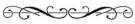

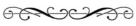

Thank you for making a difference in people's lives!

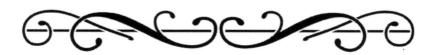

Made in the
USA
Columbia, SC